Fatimata Hassane Djibo

# Juvenile Myoclonic Epilepsy EMJ

Fatimata Hassane Djibo

# Juvenile Myoclonic Epilepsy EMJ

## Electroclinical, therapeutic and evolutionary aspects

**ScienciaScripts**

# Table of contents :

# DEDICACES

I dedicate this memoir :

**A ALLAH SOUBHANAHOU WATA ALA :**

The Clement, the Merciful, the Only One Worthy of adoration... There are no things but those that you facilitate, your slave that I am is grateful to you for having allowed her to elaborate this succinct work. I rely on you in all circumstances, it is to your power that I pity my weaknesses, for you are the strongest of supports.

I beg you to guide my steps on the paths of those you have guided, and not on the path of those you have led astray.

My God, I still need You because the road is still long and thorny, but I know that with Your support there will be no insurmountable obstacle, for only Your will is accomplished here below and in the hereafter.

To his Prophet Mohamed (peace be upon him)

**To my late father Mr HASSANE DJIBO :**

Father, you were the ideal father for us, kind, just, understanding; you taught us to love others as human beings like ourselves. You made us understand the need for effort in our work, and I'm convinced that this work is the fruit of your education.

**To my husband Mr OUSSEINI OUSMANE :**

Your patience and wisdom have helped me to overcome the most difficult situations. You are not only my husband, but also my friend and confidant. May God unite us in peace, health and longevity.

**To my mother M<sup>me</sup> HASSANE DJIBO NEE HAOUA IDE :**

Your rigorous upbringing of your children has enabled us to be where we are today. Dear mother, if today I have overcome the most difficult stages of my life, it is thanks to your education and your advice that I continue to follow; dear mother, you are my confidante, and everything for me; in all my situations I think of you. Dear mother, you have always told me that life is a box; if I do good or bad, it is on my account. Wherever I am, I try to carry out the advice you have given me. May God give us long life so that you can enjoy the fruits of the tree you planted.

**To my father, the late OUSSEINI DJIBO, my father's twin brother:**

You always wanted me to be a doctor. But unfortunately, the Almighty decided otherwise, as you passed away before I finished my studies. May your soul rest in peace.

**My beloved daughters**: Zeinab Ousseini OUSMANE and Aicha Ousseini OUSMANE. You are my comfort and my joy in life.

**To my brothers and sisters:**

The late Hamsatou Hassane Djibo, Adama H. Djibo 1, Aminata H. Djibo, Sita H. Djibo, Issoufou

H. Djibo, Mahamadou H. Djibo, Idrissa H. Djibo, Adama H. Djibo 2, Hawa H. Djibo, Mariama H. Djibo and Kadidja H. Djibo, your unconditional, material and moral support enabled me to complete this work, I dedicate this thesis to you. May God bless you all.

**To my aunt:**

$M^{me}$ Alhouseïni née Adama Ousmane: You have been a second mother to me, as well as my elementary school teacher, and you have contributed in every way to my success. May God bless you.

**To my aunts:**

Hadjo Idé, Kadi Idé, the late Hamidou Idé, Ramatou (Djiwa), Guorio: you have been my advisors, may God bless you.

**To my uncles:**

Aboubacar Ganda, Djoumassi lougua, Salifou Ousmane, Sékou Habibou Nouhou, Salifou Soffo and my nephew the late Moustapha Kadri, may the earth be light to you. Thank you for your moral and material support and for your prayers during these years of hard work. May you find in this work my most sincere thanks.

**To my brothers-in-law:**

Bouraima Seydou, the late Bouraima Saiboun Maiga, Mahamadou Tawayé and Moussa Madi, you behaved like big brothers to me. Thank you for your moral and material support. May God bless you all.

**To my cousins and nephews:**

Fatoumata .I. DJIBO my namesake, Hama Bomberi, Laila ALhousseini Thank you for your advice and prayers during these years of hard work.

**To my in-laws:** (Zalika Sékou my mother-in-law, Ousmane Joseph my father-in-law and my brothers-in-law and sisters-in-law) thank you for your support and your prayers.

**To the entire Niger community in Senegal**

Thank you for your patriotism and the moral support you have always given me.

# ACKNOWLEDGEMENTS

**Senegal** a good example of scientific research for other French-speaking African countries, not just West Africa,

It's true that the road has been long and hard, but only in the quest for knowledge, and knowledge is an inexhaustible treasure. So man's destiny is inescapable.

A welcoming land, you gave me shelter and food in your bosom. You taught me your culture without judging mine, and in your home.

And yet, I don't know what I offered you in return.

But thanks to what I've inherited from you, my doors will always be open to foreigners.

I'll represent Senegal wherever I need to; it's part of my homeland.

**To our Master, member of the jury**

**Professor Mouhamadou Mansour NDIAYE,**

Director of the Neurology DES at UCAD and chairman of our jury.

Your human qualities, your sense of responsibility, of duty and of a job well done, make you more than a teacher but an example. Your advice and pedagogical approach were a precious asset in the realization of this work.

Allow us, dear Master, to thank you most sincerely.

**To our Master, member of the jury,**

**Professor Amadou Gallo DIOP,**

Your sympathy, your simplicity, your generosity, your rigor and dedication to your work, as well as your sense of pedagogy, have won our admiration and made you a much-appreciated, esteemed and exemplary teacher.

Rest assured, dear Master, of our full gratitude.

**To our Master, member of the jury,**

**To our Master Professor Kamadore TOURE**

Your availability, your simplicity, your critical approach to scientific research and your humility make you an exemplary teacher and role model.

Rest assured, dear Master, of our full gratitude.

**To our Master and Thesis Director,**

**Professor Moustapha NDIAYE**

You opened your office door to us at every moment of the day, not only for the direction of this thesis but also for the correction of our neurological shortcomings.

Your thoroughness is a source of inspiration for every young neurologist, and I thank you for everything.

You directed the work on this dissertation with authority and scientific rigor. This work is the fruit of your efforts.

**Our masters and trainers**

Professor Massar DIAGNE

Professor Alé TIAM

Doctor-Colonel Boubou MBOUP

Professor Lala Bouna SECK,

Dr Anna Basse FAYE

Dr Adja SOW

Dr Ngore Sidi DIAGNE

Dr Marième Soda DIOP

Dr Ndeye Fatou NDOYE

Dr Mamadou SY

**To my teachers at primary, secondary and university level**

Thanks to your help, my training was a success. I am very grateful to you.

**Professor Amara CISSE,** Head of the Neurology Department at the Ngnace Deen University Hospital in Conakry, **Professor Yacouba Harouna Djimba,** lecturer at the Abdoul Moumouni Dioffo University in Niamey,

Thank you for your advice, you have contributed to my training.

**To all my colleagues**

Thank you for your help in preparing this work.

**To my friends:**

The late Rakiatou Boubacar dite Nathalie (may the earth be light to you**),** Halimatou DJIBO, Zeinab Koné, Hadiza Mounkaila Hassane, Fati Bigua Soumaïla, Maïmouna Mamoudou, Ben Adji Djibrilla, Diallo M Ibrahima, Dina, Herman, Laura, Eric, ALoise D,Maouly.F,AminatouIssoufou,Yannick,Youssouf God bless you all for the moral support you have given me.

**The Kouyaté family and Mr Assane Diouf**

Please accept the expression of my deep respect and gratitude to you...

Thank you for your efforts to integrate me into the Senegalese community.

My thanks also go to :

The administrative staff of the Faculty of Medicine, Pharmacy and Odonto-stomatology

(FMPOS) of Dakar's Cheikh Anta Diop University (UCAD)

To the teaching staff and medical and paramedical staff of the Neurology and Neurosurgery Departments of the Centre Hospitalier National Universitaire de Fann

We had a wonderful time together. Thank you for all your friendship and support.

To all those who have contributed in any way to the realization of this work. Thank you for your efforts.

# SUMMARY

**Introduction:** Juvenile myoclonic epilepsy is a form of idiopathic generalized epilepsy. It affects older children and even young adults, peaking at puberty. It usually begins between the ages of 12 and 18. Onset after the age of 30 is exceptional. The child will have one or more predominant myoclonic jerks, usually after awakening, associated or not with CGTCs and/or absences. Juvenile myoclonic epilepsy (JME) is an electro-clinical genetic epilepsy.

**Study objectives 2** Describe the electro-clinical, therapeutic and evolutionary aspects of our patients.

**Patients and method:** Our study was prospective from May 2014 to July 2015 (14-month period) at the epileptology consultation of the clinical neurophysiology department.

**Results**: There were 19 cases (11 M +9 F with a sex ratio of 1.22), mean age at onset 16.15 years, with extremes from 9 to 30. The age group most affected was 14 to 19 years, with a frequency of 36.85%. Family history of epilepsy (73.68%), consanguinity (5.26%). Myoclonic jerks associated with CGTC (64%) absences (10%). Pathological EEG in all patients. Peak-waves were most frequent (57.89%), i.e. 11 cases. PHB monotherapy was the most widely used treatment, with seizures controlled in 63.15%

(12 cases). The neurological examination was normal in all patients, with a favourable outcome in 78.45% (15 cases).

**Discussion:** Age of onset, clinical symptomatology and course are consistent with literature descriptions. However, PHB was the most commonly used molecule, contrary to the results in the literature. This may be due to its accessibility and efficacy. Wave spikes were the most frequent, which does not correspond to the results found in the literature.

This can be explained by the fact that the size of our cohort was not large and the duration of our study was not long, and also by the absence of EEG coupled with EMG. Contrary to studies found in the literature.

**Conclusion:** The characteristics of our series are similar to those of other published series in terms of age of onset, clinical symptomatology and course. Treatment and EEG do not correspond to those described in the literature. Seizures were controlled with PHB in 63.15% (12 cases).

# INTRODUCTION

Juvenile myoclonic epilepsy (JME) is a form of idiopathic generalized epilepsy (5-10% of all epilepsies), accounting for 18% of idiopathic generalized epilepsies (IGE) [3].

It's an epilepsy that affects older children and even young adults, peaking at puberty. JME is a fairly common epileptic syndrome, usually beginning in children between the ages of 12 and 18. Onset after the age of 30 remains exceptional [15].

The child will have one or more myoclonic jerks, usually after waking up [4].

Juvenile myoclonic epilepsy (JME) is also a clinically defined electro-genetic epilepsy. [3].

This definition emphasizes both the clinical and electrical aspects, requiring polygraphic recording at the very moment of the seizure.

In our context, the clinical argument has taken precedence over the electrical argument, as the majority of our patients are diagnosed on the basis of the clinic and the "intercritical" electroencephalography (EEG), which is above all "not coupled with electromyography (EMG)". And in so doing, we could be exposing our patients to an overdiagnosis of EMJ.

In this study, we propose to describe patients diagnosed with EMJ on the basis of the usual means of diagnosis used in our department.

## Study objectives

### General objective:

Describe the electro-clinical, therapeutic and evolutionary aspects of our patients

### Specific objectives :

1. Describe the semiology of seizures

2. Describe EEG abnormalities;

3. Determining treatment efficacy;

4. To determine the progressive nature of patients diagnosed with EMJ.

# I. REVIEW OF LITERATURE

**1- History**

The clinical features of JME were first described in a patient in 1867 by Herpain. In 1899, Rabot emphasized the importance and characteristics of myoclonus. In 1957, Janz and Christian reported 47 cases and proposed the name "impulsive petit mal" as a clinically definable epileptic syndrome. In the same year, Castels and Mendilaharsu in Uruguay described the features as a specific IGE syndrome. The syndrome was later called juvenile myoclonic epilepsy (de Janz) in the English language. In the same year, Castels and Mendilaharsu in Uruguay described the features as a specific IGE syndrome **[3].**

In 1989, the International League Against Epilepsy (ILAE) suggested that "Juvenile Myoclonic Epilepsy" and "Impulsive Petit Mal" were equivalent. Juvenile myoclonic epilepsy is now recognized as a common epileptic syndrome worldwide, with a large series of patients having been reported, for example, in India. [3].

**What other names are given to juvenile myoclonic epilepsy?**

Other terms used to describe juvenile myoclonic epilepsy include

- adolescent myoclonic epilepsy;

- Janz syndrome;

- Juvenile myoclonic epilepsy of Janz[4].

## 2- **Epidemiology**

Early reports favoured male predominance. The literature suggests that it generally appears in the second decade. However, the age of onset of JME covers a wide range from 8 to 36 years, with a peak onset between the ages of 12 and 18.

The incidence of JME has been estimated at 1 per 100,000 people, with a prevalence of 0.1 to 0.2 per 100,000. The prevalence of JME in large cohorts has been estimated at 5-10% of all epilepsies and 18% of idiopathic generalized epilepsies (IGE). [3].

However, EMJ cases may be less numerous in referral centers, due to the fact that most patients are easily controlled and will not be referred to specialized clinics. Thus, a lower prevalence among all epilepsy cases was reported in specialized clinics (4.3% for Janzé and 4.1% for Centon et al.) than in less selective clinics (11.4% for Wolf and Goosses, 10.7% for Obeid and Panayiotopoulos, and 10.2% for Panayiotopoulos et al. These figures were confirmed by a study from Kuala Lumpur, Malaysia: between 165 consecutive new-onset epilepsy cases. The population-based prevalence of JME, however, may be low. A study of adults (aged 15 and over) in Hong Kong found 756 cases of epilepsy, giving an epilepsy prevalence of 1.54 per thousand, including 38.7%

of idiopathic epilepsies and only 0.68% of JME cases. Mortality in JME has not been studied: JME does not appear to have a major impact on life expectancy [3].

### 3- Pathogenesis

Juvenile myoclonic epilepsy is an idiopathic generalized epilepsy syndrome with a strong genetic component. One-third to one-half of affected children have a family history of seizures or epilepsy. In some cases, children have had febrile seizures or infantile epileptic absences before developing juvenile myoclonic epilepsy.

Epilepsy is essentially genetic in origin, with a strong familial predisposition. The disease is inherited in a dominant-recessive fashion. The mutation in question has been identified in the gene **[6]**.

In rare cases, children with juvenile myoclonic epilepsy also have structural abnormalities in the brain, but this does not appear to affect response to treatment or outlook. One MRI study found that people with juvenile myoclonic epilepsy and other idiopathic generalized epilepsies had subtle differences in gray matter volume, gray matter distribution and brain metabolism compared with people without idiopathic generalized epilepsy [4].

## 4- Clinical and paraclinical

### Clinic

It's a primary, generalized epilepsy, beginning around puberty and manifested by isolated or repeated bilateral myoclonic jerks, usually affecting the upper limbs, particularly frequent in the morning after waking up, tonicoclonic generalized seizures and absences. But myoclonic jerks are the most frequent. Lack of sleep, particularly irregular sleep patterns, stimulants of any kind (alcohol, drugs, etc.), menstruation, stress and strong emotions, all favour myoclonus. Development and neurological examination are normal [4].

### Paraclinical

Patients with EMJ have an intercritical tracing that may be normal or show generalized, asymptomatic polypointer or polypointer-wave puffs. During a myoclonic seizure, the EEG shows bilateral, synchronous bursts of 3.5Hz peak waves or poly-peak waves, or very high-frequency poly-peak waves. EEG discharges are often longer than the seizure itself. There are various provocation methods for recording pathological brain electrical activity:

1) perform a night EEG, 2) induce hyperventilation due to sleep deprivation,

3) light stimuli can sometimes trigger attacks. Photosensitivity is more age-related. It develops between the ages of 10 and 15 and resolves around the age of 20.

## 5- Treatment basics

Juvenile myoclonic epilepsy is easily controlled with medication and lifestyle adjustments. In fact, over 80% of patients manage to control their epilepsy. Treatment leads to the disappearance of myoclonus and photosensitivity, which diminish spontaneously over the course of the third decade. Discontinuation of treatment, often attempted after several seizure-free years under treatment, is followed by a recurrence of seizures in more than half of cases, especially when people deviate from a healthy, regular lifestyle [1].

Response to treatment is brilliant (Valproate, clonazepam). JME is drug-dependent: in 90% of cases, discontinuation of treatment leads to a recurrence of clinical manifestations. Treatment must therefore be continued for a very long time, sometimes for life. [15].

Phenobarbital can also be used in cases of myoclonus when there is no association with absences.

# II.  PATIENTS AND METHOD

### 1.  Study framework :

This study was carried out in the neurology department of the CHU Faim in Dakar, Senegal. The department has a triple vocation: patient care, training in neuroscience and research into neurological disorders.

### 2.  Type of study

This is a cross-sectional, prospective descriptive study of a series of nineteen cases of juvenile myoclonic epilepsy in consultation at the neurology department of the Centre Hospitalier et Universitaire de Faim in Dakar between May 2014 and July 2015.

### 3.  Population

Children (girls and boys) consulting the neurology department for epileptiform and/or epileptic seizures were included during our study period.

### 4.  Inclusion criteria:

- All patients reporting myoclonic seizures,
- Intercritical EEG with arguments in favor of epileptic disease

- And patient labeled known to suffer from JME.

## 5. Non-inclusion criteria:

- All patients meeting the inclusion criteria, but with a serious and/or acute pathology requiring urgent care or rigorous monitoring.

## 6. Equipment:

To carry out our study, we had at our disposal :

- Patient files,

- Survey sheets designed for this purpose

## 7. Variables :

In our study, the following variables were analyzed:

- Age of onset

- Family history of epilepsy and consanguinity

- The semiology of myoclonic seizures,

- Frequency of attacks,

- Electrical faults at the time of diagnosis,

- The treatment taken by each patient and

- Post-therapeutic electro-clinical evolution.

## 8. Limitations:

The limitations of our study were the absence of EEG coupled with EMG

## 9. Statistical analysis :

Data were entered into SPSS version 16 for Windows. We performed univariate analyses (calculation of frequencies, means and standard deviations). We then compared electro-clinical profiles before and after treatment.

## 10. Ethical considerations :

Patients were selected after obtaining informed consent from their parents and/or guardians regarding the general purpose of the study.

# III. RESULTS: OBSERVATIONS

We report the observations of nineteen patients seen in epileptology consultation at the Fann clinical neurophysiology department.

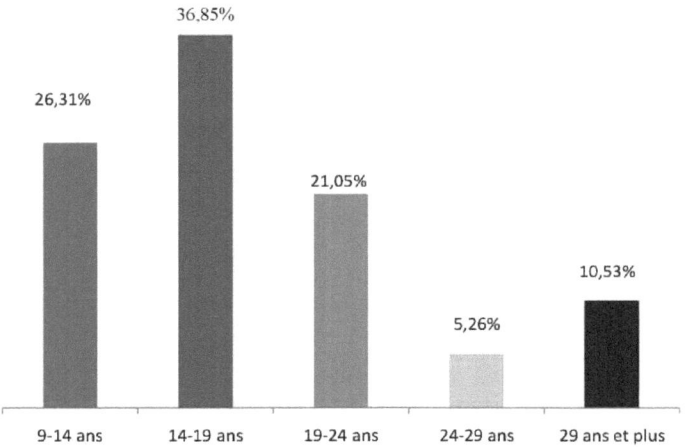

**Figure 1: Age distribution of patients**

Our patients were divided into 5 age groups, with extremes ranging from 9 to 30 years. The age group most affected was 14 to 19, with a frequency of 36.85%.

**Table I: Distribution of patients by gender**

| Gender | Number of patients | Percentage (%) |
|--------|--------------------|----------------|
| Male   | 11                 | 57 ,89         |
| Female | 8                  | 42,11          |
| Total  | 19                 | 100            |

Our study included both sexes, in search of a predominance. Men were more

affected than women, with 11 cases (57.89) and a sex ratio of 1.22.

**Table II Distribution of patients according to history**

| History | Number of patients | Percentage(%) |
|---------|--------------------|----------------|
| **Familial epilepsy** |  |  |
| Yes | 14 | 73,68 |
| No | 5 | 26,32 |
| **Parental consanguinity** |  |  |
| Yes | 01 | 5,26 |
| No | 18 | 94,74 |

We found a family history in 73.68% of patients, and parental consanguinity in

5.26%.

**Table III :: Distribution of patients according to clinical aspects**

| Clinical aspects | Number of patients | Percentage(%) |
|---|---|---|
| **Age of onset** | | |
| <9 | 2 | 10,52 |
| 9-19 | 12 | 63,16 |
| 19-29 | 3 | 15,80 |
| 29 and over | 2 | 10,52 |
| **Epileptic manifestations** | | |
| Isolated myoclonus | 3 | 15,80 |
| Myoclonus and CGTC | 9 | 47,37 |
| Myoclonus and Absence | 5 | 26,30 |
| Myoclonus +CGTC+Absence | 2 | 10,53 |
| **Neurological examination** Normal | 19 | 100 |

The mean age of onset was 16.15 years. 10.52% of patients had their seizures before the age of 9, 63.16% between the ages of 9 and 19, 15.80% between the ages of 19 and 29, and 10.52% after the age of 29.

Our study focused on the type of seizure, the clinic was predominated by muscle twitches or 100% but with an association or not to other types of seizures (CGTC, absence or isolated myoclonus):

9 cases of CGTC, i.e. 47.66%, followed by absences with 5 cases, i.e. 26.31%, including 2 cases of myoclonus associated with CGTC and absence, and 3 cases of myoclonus without association with other seizure types.

Among the 9 cases of myoclonus, we have 7 cases of myoclonus on awakening, 1 case of myoclonus triggered by writing, and one case of myoclonus triggered by emotions.

Seizures are triggered by lack of sleep, stimulants, stress and strong emotions, and predominate in the upper limbs. Neurological examination was normal in all patients.

**Table IV: Distribution of patients according to EEG type and results:**

| EEG results | Number of patients | Percentage(%) |
|---|---|---|
| **Sleep EEG** | | |
| Wave polytips | 01 | 5,26 |
| Peak wave flushes | 02 | 10,52 |
| Wave and polytips waves | 01 | 5,26 |
| **EEG sleep and wake-up** | 01 | 5,26 |
| **Standby EEG** | | |
| Peak Wave Flushes | 09 | 47,37 |

| Generalized | | |
|---|---|---|
| Wave polytips | 04 | 21,05 |
| Wave and Wave polytips | 03 | 15,80 |
| No anomaly | 01 | 5,26 |
| Diffuse slowdown | 01 | 5 ,26 |

---

Sleep EEG was performed in 4 patients, showing 10.52% spike waves (2 cases), 5.26% polypoints (1 case) and 5.26% a combination of spike waves and polypoints (1 case). Among the 4 cases, there were 5.26% puffs, i.e. one case on awakening.

The waking EEG was performed in 18 patients, of whom 47.37% had wave spikes (9 cases), 21.05% had wave polypoints (4 cases) and 15.80% had a combination of wave spikes and polypoints. The waking EEG was normal, but showed abnormalities during sleep: 5.26% had diffuse slowing (one case).

A total of 26.31% of polypointes ondes during wakefulness and sleep, i.e. 5 cases, 21.06% of the combination of polypointes and pointes ondes during wakefulness, i.e. 4 cases, and 57.89% of pointes ondes during wakefulness and sleep, i.e. 11 cases.

**OBSERVATION 1**

A 16-year-old female Senegalese student was seen in consultation at the epileptology clinic for myoclonus in the neurophysiology department of CHNU de Fann in July 2014. The neurological examination was normal.

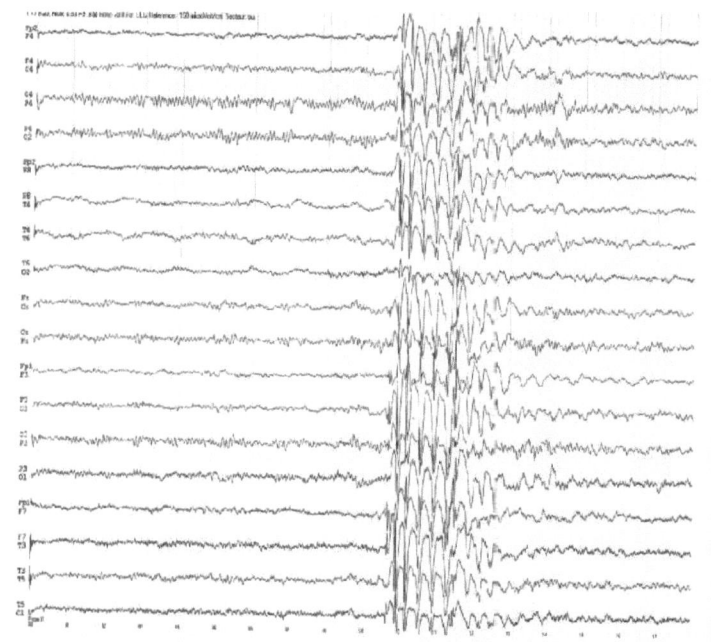

<u>**Figure 2**</u>: **Standby EEG**

The patient's waking EEG showed background activity with an alpha rhythm of 11c /sec, posterior, symmetrical, synchronous and reactive. Generalized wave spikes predominated in the bifrontal region. HPN and SLI had no effect.

The patient was treated with phenobarbital at a dose of 100mg per day. The evolution was favorable, with seizures disappearing for 12 months. But returned on July 2, 2015 for myoclonus triggered by therapeutic discontinuation.

## OBSERVATION 2

A 16-year-old patient received in epiletology consultation at the neurophysiology department of CHNU de Fann for epileptic seizures with loss of consciousness since 2010. 2 years ago, generalized myoclonus on awakening and at the time of the seizures increased in the picture. Neurological examination returned normal. Her sister has seizures.

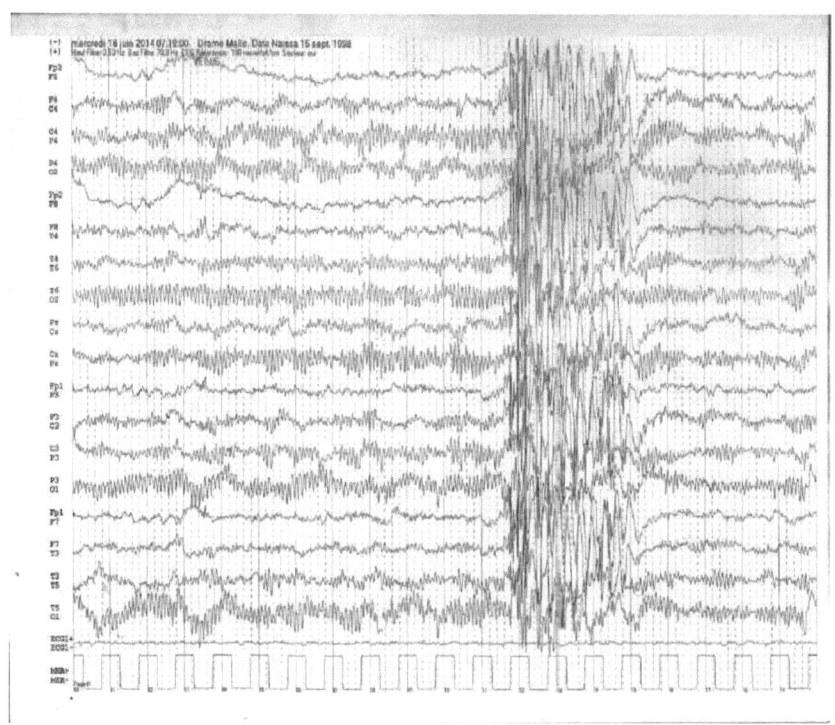

**Figure 3: Standby EEG**

The waking EEG showed an Alpha rhythm at 8-9 cycles/second, posterior, well modulated, bilateral, symmetrical, synchronous and reactive. There were also numerous 3-second bursts of poorly drawn, diffuse peak waves, strongly activated during drowsiness, totally subclinical. The EEG shows idiopathic generalized epilepsy of the EMJ type.

The patient was put on sodium valproate at a dose of 40 mg/kg/d in 2 doses. The evolution was favorable, with disappearance of the seizures.

## OBSERVATION 3

A 23-year-old Senegalese student patient, was received in epileptology consultation at the neurophysiology department of CHNU de Fann on May 27, 2014 for myoclonus that lasted two years, beginning in the left lower limb, then generalizing, and these myoclonus are triggered in situations of nervousness, shouting , excessive speech and fatigue. He had seizures once or twice a week. There was a family history of seizures in an aunt. Neurological examination came back normal.

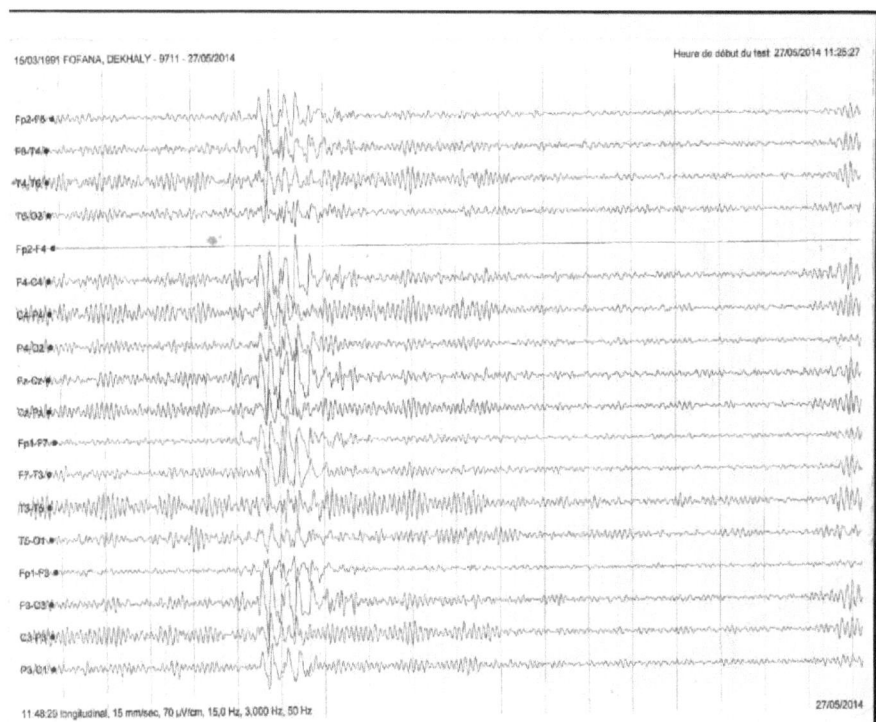

**Figure 4: Standby EEG**

The patient's waking EEG showed background activity with a 9-10 Hz alpha rhythm that was bilateral, symmetrical, synchronous and reactive to eye closure and opening. There was a generalized spike-wave flush at the start of the recording, which was repeated at the end of intermittent light stimulation. Hyperventilation had no effect.

The patient was treated with phenobarbital at a dose of 100mg daily. The evolution was favorable, with disappearance of the seizures.

**Table V: Distribution of patients according to treatment**

| Treatment | Number of patientsPercentage | (%) |
|-----------|------------------------------|-----|
| PHB | 1263 | ,15 |
| VPA | 736 | ,85 |
| Total | | 19100 |

All patients received appropriate medical treatment, with seizures controlled by

monotherapy with phenobarbital or sodium valpoate. Phenobarbital was the most

commonly used molecule, in 12 cases (63.15%), followed by VPA in 7 cases

(36.84%).

**Table VI: Distribution of patients according to progress**

| Evolution | Number of patients | Percentage (%) |
|-----------|--------------------|----------------|
| Favorable | 15 | 78,95 |
| Unfavorable | 04 | 21,05 |
| Total | 19 | 100 |

We found a favorable outcome in 78.95% (15 cases) and an unfavorable outcome in

21.05% (4 cases).

# IV.   DISCUSSION

JME is defined by the absence of an acquired history that could explain the seizures. It is an epilepsy of essentially genetic origin, with a strong familial predisposition. We considered a family history to be any case of epilepsy in a relative of the patient, whether a direct ascendant, a collateral (brother or sister) or a distant relative. Thus, we found that 14 of the 19 cases (73.68%) had a family history of epilepsy, and one case (5.26%) had parental consanguinity. This comes close to the results put forward by those who say that a third to half of affected children have a family history of seizures or epilepsy [6].

Our patients were divided into 5 age groups, with extremes ranging from 9 to 30 years. The most affected age group was 14 to 19 years, with a frequency of 36.85%. The literature suggests that JME generally appears in the second decade. However, the age of onset of JME covers a wide range from 8 to 36 years, with peak onset between 12 and 18 years [3], which is close to our results. The mean age of onset was 16.15 years. 10.52% of patients had their attacks before the age of 9, 63.16% between the ages of 9 and 19, 15.80% between 19 and 29 and 10.52% of cases after the age of 29, which is in line with the results reported by others who say that the age of onset of JME covers a wide range from 8 to 36 years, with a peak onset between 12 and 18[3] .

The incidence of JME has been estimated at 1 per 100,000 people, with a prevalence of 0.1 to 0.2 per 100,000. The prevalence of JME in large cohorts has been estimated at 5-10% of all epilepsies and 18% of idiopathic generalized epilepsies (IGE).

Our study included both sexes in search of a predominance. Men were more affected than women, with 11 cases (57.89%) versus 8 cases (42.10%). Our results corroborate those of Carlos, who states that early reports were in favor of male predominance.

Our study focused on the type of seizure, the clinic was predominated by muscle twitches or 100% but with an association or not to other types of seizures (CGTC, absence or pure myoclonus):

9 cases of CGTC, i.e. 47.66%, followed by absences with 5 cases, i.e. 26.31%, including 2 cases of myoclonus associated with CGTC and absences and 3 cases of isolated myoclonus without CGTC.

association with other types of seizures. Among the 9 cases of myoclonus, we have 7 cases of myoclonus on awakening, 1 case of myoclonus triggered by writing and by emotions.

Seizures are triggered by lack of sleep, stimulants, stress and strong emotions, and predominate in the upper limbs. Development and neurological examination are normal.

Our results corroborate those reported in the literature, which state that JME manifests itself as isolated or repeated bilateral myoclonic jerks, most often affecting the upper limbs, particularly frequent in the morning after waking up, tonicoclonic generalized seizures and absences. But myoclonic jerks are the most frequent. Lack of sleep, particularly irregular sleep patterns, stimulants of any kind (alcohol, drugs, etc.), menstruation, stress and strong emotions, all favour myoclonus. Development and neurological examination are normal. [4]

Our patients underwent EEG and the tracings showed epileptic abnormalities. Our results corroborate those reported in the literature, which state that juvenile myoclonic epilepsy (JME) is an electroclinical genetic epilepsy [3].

The patients presented with intercritical epileptic discharges (PPO and irregular, generalized rapid point-waves), especially at SLI and HPN. Our results corroborate those found by Elizabeth et al [4]. The most characteristic epileptic discharge was the spike-wave complex, which does not correspond to the results found in other studies. This may be explained by the fact that the size of our cohort was not large and the duration of our study was not long, unlike studies found in the literature.

All patients received appropriate medical treatment, and monotherapy with phenobarbital or sodium valproate enabled seizures to be controlled. Phenobarbital was the most commonly used molecule, in 12 cases or 63.15%, followed by VPA in 7 cases or 36.84%, which does not corroborate those who say that his patients were able to achieve seizure control in 78.9% on Sodium Valproate and the remainder on Phenobarbital [2].

This is due not only to the efficacy of Phenobarbital on myoclonus, but also to its affordability compared with sodium Valproate. But there can often be persistence under treatment, which may be due either to poor lifestyle habits, poor compliance or the use of inappropriate molecules such as Carbamazepine.

Apart from everything else, sodium valpoate, phenobarbital and benzodiazepines are currently the most effective drugs for treating JME [2].

Phenobarbital is not used in cases of JME where there is an association with absences. [15]

All our patients had a favourable outcome at the start of treatment, but subsequently, due to poor compliance and lack of hygiene, seizures reappeared in 4 patients (21.05%), including two students and two pupils. Seizures reappeared mainly during examinations, following sleep deprivation or the use of stimulants, or when medication was interrupted.

Our results corroborate those reported in the literature that juvenile myoclonic epilepsy is easily controlled with drug treatment and lifestyle adjustment. In fact, over 80% of patients manage to control their epilepsy. Treatment leads to the disappearance of myoclonus and photosensitivity, which diminish spontaneously over the course of the third decade. Discontinuation of treatment, often attempted after several seizure-free years under treatment, is followed by a recurrence of seizures in more than half the cases, especially when people deviate from a healthy, regular lifestyle [1].

# CONCLUSION

The characteristics of our series are similar to those of other published series, in terms of age of onset, sex, clinical symptomatology and course. The electroencephalography (EEG) and treatment did not correspond to those described in the literature. A family history of epilepsy was present in the majority of cases. Response to treatment with phenobarbital monotherapy resulted in seizure control in the majority of cases. We have noted that seizures attempt to reappear with poor compliance and lifestyle habits. Juvenile myoclonic epilepsy is pharmacosensitive and pharmacodependent.

# REFERENCES

1-BOUGTEBA.A, BASSIR.A, BELAIDI.H, BROOK.N, LAHJOUJI .F, KABLY.B.

Clinical and electroencephalographic aspects of juvenile myoclonic epilepsy:

Study of 122 cases. Service de Neurophysiologie Clinique. Specialty Hospital,

Rabat, Morocco. Revue maghrébine de neurosciences 2009.

2- Betul Baykan, Iris E. Martinez-Juarez, Ebru A. Altindag, Carol S. Camfield, Peter

R.Camfield. Lifetime prognosis of juvenile myoclonic epilepsy. Epilepsy and

behavior 28(2013) S18-S24

3- Carol S.Camfield, Pasquale Striano, Peter R.Canfield. Epidemiology of juvenile

myoclonic epilepsy. Epilepsy and behavior 28(2013) S15-S17

4- Elizabeth J. Donner, MD, FRCPC 2/4/2010 Documentation / Epilepsy /

Understanding epilepsy and its diagnosis /Epilepsy syndromes accessed

15/07/2014

5- Cassim .F, E.Houdayer. Neurophysiology of myoclonus. Clinical Neurophysiology

36 (2006) 281-291

6- Dr Gérard Emmerich. Epilepsy and treatment *16/11/201108:25:27, Encyclopedias, accessed 15/07/2014*

7- Rubboli.G, Tassinari. C.A. Negative myoclonus: An overview of its clinical features, pathophysiological mechanism and management. Clinical Neurophysiology 36 (2006) 337-343

8- Cuvellier.JC, Lamblin .MD, Cuisset.JM, Vallée.L,k, Nuyts.JP. Reflex benign myoclonic epilepsy of the infant. Arch pediatr 1997; 4:755-758

9- John N Caviness ,Peter Brown. Myoclonus: Current concepts and recent advances. Lancet neurol 2004; 3:598-607

10- Joke M Dijk, Marina AJ Tijssen. Management of patients with myoclonus: Available therapies and the need for an evidence-based-approach. Lancet Neurol 2010; 9:1028-36

11-Jonathan Carr. Classifying myoclonus: Riddle, wrapped in a mystery, inside an enigma: Parkinsonism and related disorder. *Division of Neurology, Faculty of Health Sciences, University of Stellenbosch, South Africa*, 18S1 (2012) S174-S176

12-Vercueil.L, Krieger.J, Les myoclonies chez l'adulte: démarche diagnostique.

*Service de neurologie, Hôpitaux universitaires de Grenoble ,*NeurophysiolClin

2001 ; 31 :3-17


13-  Borg M. Symptomatic myoclonus. Clinical Neurophysiology 36(2006) 309-318


14-  P.Genton. Unverricht-Lundborg disease. Revuneurol (Paris) 2006;162:8-9,819-

826


15-  P.Thomas, A.Arzimanoglou. Epilepsies 3rd edition Paris, Masson

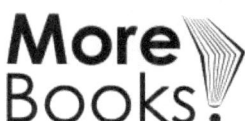
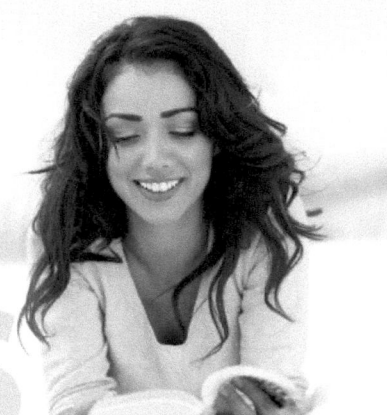

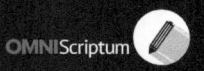

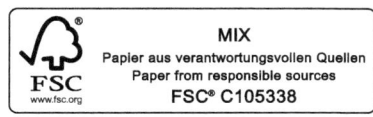
Printed by Books on Demand GmbH, Norderstedt / Germany